Keeping It Off!

The Last Diet Book You'll Ever Need

Marie M. Barbieri

LONGMEADOW PRESS

This book is intended as a reference volume only, not as a medical manual or guide to self-treatment. It is not intended as a substitute for the medical advice of physicians. The reader should regularly consult a physician in general, and particularly for any symptoms. If you suspect that you have a medical problem, we urge you to seek competent medical help. Keep in mind that exercise and nutritional need vary from person to person, depending on age, sex, health status and individual variations. The information here is intended to help you make informed decisions about your health, not as a substitute for any treatment that may have been prescribed by your doctor.

Published by Longmeadow Press, 201 High Ridge Road, Stamford, CT 06904.

Cover and interior design by Barbara Cohen Aronica.

ISBN: 0-681-40984-3

PRINTED IN THE UNITED STATES OF AMERICA

0 9 8 7 6 5 4 3 2 1

To *my* true family . . .

FOREWORD

Over the past twenty-five years, in my work as a university professor, counselor and human relations consultant, I have used a variety of methods to help students and clients tap into their inner resources to achieve personal and academic growth. Motivating indivduals to look for positive ways of learning and growing is exciting and rewarding. **Keeping It Off!** is a fine example of good, positive motivational techniques and an invaluable tool for those who have set weight loss goals they not only intend to reach, but to maintain for life.

For the many who struggle with weight problems, the real challenge lies in keeping the pounds off once they have been lost. **Keeping It Off!** cuts to the heart of this problem. In brief, clear language, Ms. Barbieri has provided a model of positive thinking and positive planning for graduates of any diet program who want to maintain a chosen weight. The book not only provides guidelines and directives but many new ideas and choices that make weight maintenance feasible and enjoyable.

In addition, the ideas and concepts in this book serve as a metaphor for anyone who sets goals of any kind and is determined, through positive habits and routines, to continue along successful paths. The author, who has walked in the shoes of an overweight person, honestly and sympathetically identifies with the trials and pitfalls of those who wrestle with self-direction and control in their everyday lives.

So, continue to be a winner—a person who is always on a journey toward a goal. By planning and following the thoughtful, creative suggestions and routines presented in this concise, well written book, you are on your way to life-long success.

Enjoy keeping it off!

Gerald M. Arndt, Ed.D
Professor, University of Bridgeport
Human Relations Consultant and Therapist

About the Author

In 1960 Marie M. Barbieri was a size 14. In less than a year she was down to a size 9 and continued dieting until she became a 5. Marie is still a size 5 today, and her program of weight maintenance has been the basis of her successful diet counseling practice. A graduate of Trinity College, Washington, D.C. with a minor in Education, she holds a Master's degree in Counseling from the University of Bridgeport. She has been a behavioral counselor for six years.

"You, heavy? Never!"

I deliberately destroyed a photograph of myself—taken when I was eight years old. This photo had become a too painful reminder of my childhood, when I was "pleasingly plump." Actually, I was fat. I weighed over one hundred pounds and I was four feet tall.

I could tell you I doused this infamous photograph with kerosene, igniting it at sunset as a symbolic act of mid-life renewal. Instead, I merely tore my picture into uneven fragments and shoved them into the kitchen garbage. *This* was truly symbolic! From that moment I felt a new determination to control my weight for all time!

Keeping It Off! describes a maintenance system that gradually emerged as I struggled to simplify my eating life. Static ideas about food and drink were replaced with a dynamic method for controlling calories. By adapting my eating and drinking habits to fit my lifestyle changes, I discovered an exciting system for regulating my weight on an ongoing basis. The perennial question for most dieters—"How do I keep my weight off?"—was now answered. I was able to keep the weight off by recording what I ate and drank, one day at a time. *Controlled eating became a part of my daily life, not only a part of my weight-loss program.*

Over the past fifteen years, I have maintained a weight level and eating style that look and feel good for me. Truly, one of my fondest experiences is to hear people remark: "You, heavy? Never!" I too find it hard to believe. My slim self-image is the only picture I plan to see for the rest of my life.

Diet is a four-letter word!

The word *diet* suggests everything that is negative: deprivation, denial, disgust with oneself. The word *diet* traditionally describes a general discomfort which continues for a temporary period, only to be repeated at a later time after the weight is gained back.

A more dynamic concept of *diet* is *weight management. Weight management* means an effective change in everyday eating habits that is enjoyable and beneficial. *Weight management* implies control; suggests a sense of direction, an attitude that evolves with *your* personal life. Because you make day-to-day decisions, a flexibility develops that enables you to alter your approach toward food. More beneficial ways of eating gradually replace ineffective habits and beliefs.

Gone are the "guilts." You put far behind you thoughts of eating the "wrong" foods. "Temptation" becomes a term of the past. You discover a new freedom to choose—a new freedom to lose, gain, or maintain weight. Within this flexible framework you rediscover one of the basic pleasures of life. *Food is a basic pleasure,* not a "compulsion" or an "addiction."

Losing excess weight is an initially challenging task. You gradually replace old fashioned dieting with your newly developed skills of *weight management.* Denial becomes a discarded part of your past. *Directed eating becomes a permanent practice of your life. Directed eating heartily affirms that "eating to live" is a delight!*

Keeping It Off! . . . is a "maintenance manual" that talks to you about changing your eating habits. *You* change the way you talk to yourself about food, about eating. *You* change the *way* you eat. *You* feel good, *you* look good, *you change your life!!*

I

New Thoughts About Old Ideas

◆ • ◆ • ◆ • ◆ • ◆ • ◆ • ◆ • ◆ • ◆ • ◆ • ◆ • ◆ • ◆ • ◆ • ◆ • ◆ • ◆ • ◆ • ◆

Once there was an experienced dieter. *S/he followed a doctor-approved diet faithfully (well, almost) and succeeded in losing the desired weight. And when s/he returned to everyday eating, s/he discovered a better way to maintain weight: S/he changed his or her eating habits.*

◆ • ◆ • ◆ • ◆ • ◆ • ◆ • ◆ • ◆ • ◆ • ◆ • ◆ • ◆ • ◆ • ◆ • ◆ • ◆ • ◆ • ◆ • ◆

The ***experienced dieter*** plans . . .

REFOCUSING

We are always on a diet.
We traditionally understand *diet* as a weight-loss program.
Webster defines *diet* in broader terms:

> "1. Habitual course of living or especially, feeding; hence, food and drink regularly provided or consumed; fare. 2. Prescribed allowance of food with reference to a particular state of health; regimes prescribed."

Diet is a weight management program. By consciously choosing food and drink along with (routine) physical activity, a person can lose, gain, or maintain weight. *Diet* is the quantity and quality of food and drink you consume from day to day.

A *diet* is a food management program which you *choose* to control your weight:

You can lose weight.
(Your weight-loss diet is temporary or you would disappear.)
You can gain weight.
(Sometimes people need to!)
You can maintain weight.
(Your weight-maintenance diet is flexible.)

Weight management = food management + drink management + *physical activity.*

Controlled weight management produces more satisfaction . . .
Effective weight management produces day-to-day satisfaction.

Choose a diet—any diet that your doctor approves.
Choose a diet—that meets your body's needs.
Choose a diet—that matches your lifestyle.

You may choose a weight-loss diet. (Usually.)
You may choose a weight-gain diet. (Occasionally.)
You may choose a weight-maintenance diet. (Ideally.)

A weight-loss diet is temporary.
There are forbidden foods & drinks.
There is controlled eating.

A maintenance diet is ongoing.
All foods and drinks are legal.
There is controlled eating.

Controlled eating is part of all diets: a weight-loss diet
a weight-gain diet
a weight-maintenance diet.

Food selection and portion size are the control factors in any diet.

Controlled eating is directed eating.
Controlled eating is not deprived eating.
Controlled eating is the eating you choose.
Controlled eating feels good!

Controlled eating is part of weight loss, part of weight gain, and part of weight maintenance.

FOOD SELECTION

". . . the foods you choose . . ."

The foods you choose determine your weight management program:
Low calorie foods usually result in weight loss or weight maintenance.
High calorie foods usually result in weight gain.

High calorie foods are usually forbidden on a weight-loss diet.
High calorie foods are legal on a weight-gain or weight maintenance diet.

(Occasionally, high calorie foods are permitted on a weight-loss diet. You can **TAKE A TASTE!**)

Conscious *portion control* legalizes your eating of high calorie foods.
You *can* eat high calorie foods on your maintenance diet.
You *can* eat high calorie foods on your weight-loss diet, occasionally.

You choose the portions.
You choose the calories.
You choose your weight.

You choose the foods you eat.
You choose the quantity of food you eat.
You choose the quality of food you eat.
You choose your eating style!

Controlled eating is not only a part of weight loss . . .
Controlled eating is a part of maintenance!
Controlled eating is part of life . . .
Controlled eating is a way of life!

Controlled eating is a part of parties!
Controlled eating is a part of restaurants!
Controlled eating is a part of holidays!

Controlled eating is a part of birthdays!
Controlled eating is a part of anniversaries!
Controlled eating is a part of family reunions!

Controlled eating is a part of business luncheons!
Controlled eating is a part of vacations
Controlled eating is a part of life!

Controlled eating is a way of life !. . .

You make the choices . . .
You look the way you want to look . . .
You feel the way you want to feel . . .
You control your life!

Your life is pleasurable . . . . your life is enjoyable!

PORTION CONTROL

". . . the amount of food you choose . . ."

Traditionally, we associate *diet* with deprivation, forbidden foods, external control. When we do this, we are actually noting the temporary aspects of a weight-loss program. Once the excess weight is lost, deprivation becomes direction, forbidden becomes legal.

The bridge between a weight-loss diet and a maintenance diet is

PORTION CONTROL

is part of a day-to-day weight-maintenance program.

What do a weight-loss diet, a weight-gain diet, and a maintenance diet have in common?

PORTION CONTROL

PORTION CONTROL

A weight-loss diet defines portions.
A weight-gain diet defines portions.
A maintenance diet defines portions.

Consciously measuring food "measures" calories.
Consciously measuring food controls calories.
Consciously measuring food establishes

PORTION CONTROL

Your weight-loss diet defines portions.
Your maintenance diet defines portions.
Your maintenance diet re-defines self-control.

PORTION CONTROL is established when you become aware (routinely) of the types and amounts of food you eat . . .

You select a combination of foods.
You choose portions for calorie control.
You choose portions for quality.

PORTION CONTROL directs my eating . . . I modify my eating habits while I lose weight.

While I lose weight I can TAKE A TASTE of high-calorie foods.
When I TAKE A TASTE I enhance my eating.
When I TAKE A TASTE I control my eating.

TAKE A TASTE

IS

PORTION CONTROL

When I use PORTION CONTROL I direct my eating . . .
I continue to modify my eating habits
after I lose the weight.

Larger portions of low calorie foods have become
the bulk of my eating.

I sometimes eat modified portions of my favorite
high calorie foods.
Sometimes I "TAKE A TASTE" . . .
Sometimes I split a dessert . . .

On a maintenance diet all foods are legal.

When I use

FOOD SELECTION

plus

PORTION CONTROL

I direct my eating!

ACTIVITY LEVEL

". . . the activities you choose . . ."

Please add your own suggestions to this partial list:

- take a walk
- ride a (stationary) bicycle
- do aerobics
- climb up and down stairs
- chase a squirrel
- chase your boyfriend
- chase your wife
- jog
- run away from your girlfriend
- run away from your husband
- dig a ditch
- mine gold in a gold mine
- climb a mountain
- climb a wall
- climb into bed
- climb on board

Use your Imagination!

FOOD SELECTION

PORTION CONTROL

ACTIVITY LEVEL

THE BUILDING BLOCKS
OF
WEIGHT MANAGEMENT

The building blocks of maintenance . . .

SPECIAL REFOCUSING

You eat, you don't cheat . . .
    You don't cheat, you eat . . .

You choose, you don't cheat . . .
    You don't cheat, you choose . . .

You choose to eat . . .
    The kind of food you eat
    The amount of food you eat
        Produces a result: weight loss
                                   weight gain
                                   weight maintenance.

I **CHOOSE**, I DO NOT CHEAT.
I CANNOT CHEAT MYSELF.
I CANNOT FOOL MYSELF.
I CHOOSE TO TAKE CONTROL!

Large portions of low calorie foods become the bulk of my eating . . .
Small portions of high calorie foods enhance the bulk of my eating.

"Half a portion of high calorie foods is better than none."

When you find an ad on television that simply declares:

"WEIGHT CONTROL IS PORTION CONTROL!"

. . . then you're going to witness a new beginning . . .

This maintenance manual can help you begin your new life!

This maintenance manual is designed for the experienced dieter!

♦ • ♦ • ♦ • ♦ • ♦ • ♦ • ♦ • ♦ • ♦ • ♦ • ♦ • ♦ • ♦ • ♦ • ♦ • ♦ • ♦ • ♦ • ♦

The experienced dieter discovers . . .

FOOD SELECTION

PORTION CONTROL

ACTIVITY LEVEL

. . . are the building blocks of weight maintenance!

II

Awareness–You're in Control

Once there was an effective dieter. *S/he decided that once the weight was lost, there were no forbidden foods. And when s/he returned to everyday eating, s/he discovered gaining a few pounds was no longer a trigger for overeating: s/he successfully changed his or her eating beliefs.*

The ***effective dieter*** plans . . .

REFOCUSING

Observe your eating patterns for at least a month . . .

Keep a daily record of everything you eat, and when you eat it. Also, what you drink, and when you drink it.

How often do you like to eat and drink?
Three times a day?
More often or less?
Regular size portions, or mini-meals?

Are you usually away at lunch time?

Do you spend most of your eating time at home?

Are restaurants part of your lifestyle?

Do you entertain frequently?

The answers to these questions will help you design a successful weight management program which accommodates your special needs. By increasing your awareness, you can design a food management program to be used for all times. Your awareness will increase daily.

List all foods and drinks you consume each day, immediately after you eat and/or drink. *Include all snacks, nibbles and tastes.* Be specific.

On arising:	large glass of water
Breakfast:	4 oz. orange juice ½ cup oatmeal with whole milk coffee, black
Coffee, break:	coffee black ½ donut
Lunch:	½ tuna salad sandwich diet soda five potato chips (left rest)
Afternoon:	1 large apple 1 small candy bar, chocolate
Dinner:	3 medium slices turkey, white meat ½ cup stuffing ½ cup broccoli small dish jello (diet) wine spritzer (club soda with large splash of wine)
Evening:	herbal tea, orange 3 small chocolate chip cookies

This growing awareness will give you more control over your eating behavior. Self-directed eating and drinking will become a more conscious part of your everyday life.

Design your own eating profile.

Start with your *family eating style.*

Then add your personal eating style.

Finally consider your eating lifestyle.

IDENTIFY YOUR FAMILY EATING STYLE

Does your family celebrate sweets? ______

Does your family "love" pizza and breads? ______

Does your family "live to eat" or love to eat? ______

Does your family eat very large portions? ______

Does your family call large portions normal-size? ______

Does your family eat mini-portions? ______

Does your family nibble? ______

Does your family nibble all day? ______

Do you cook for your family? ______

Does your family cook for you? ______

Write down any other thoughts that come to you about your *family eating style.* ____________________

____

____

Eating patterns are learned . . .
Food preferences are learned.

Be kind to your *family eating style.*
Pay attention to it . . .
Respect it . . .

Once upon a time there was a family who ate olives only on holidays. Grandmother would put a large earthenware bowl of black olives in the center of the dining room table every Easter, every Thanksgiving, every Christmas, *every* holiday! Within minutes the olives would disappear. Year after year this would happen. Until finally, last year, each member of the family decided to bring his or her own can of olives.

Eating patterns are learned . . .
Food *preferences are learned . . .*

IDENTIFY YOUR PERSONAL EATING STYLE

What are your favorite foods?______________________________

____

What food(s) *must* you eat?_______________________________

____

What food(s) can you do without?__________________________

____

How much food do you have to eat?_________________________

____

Do you eat mini-portions?________________________________

Do you eat large portions?_______________________________

Do you nibble all day?___________________________________

What foods "turn you on" at parties_________________________

____

What food(s) *must* you have at parties?______________________

____

Eating patterns are learned . . .
Food preferences are learned.

IDENTIFY YOUR EATING LIFESTYLE

Do you eat out often?____________________

Do you eat at restaurants?____________________

Do you eat at fast food places?____________________

Do you entertain often?____________________

At home?____________________

At restaurants?____________________

Are you a marathon runner?____________________

Do you eat "on the run?"____________________

Do you prefer quiet, leisurely meals?____________________

Are quiet, leisurely meals even possible?____________________

Do you eat most of your meals at home?____________________

Does this make you happy or sad?____________________

Can you think of any changes you *might* want to make?__________

Eating patterns are learned . . .
Food preferences are learned.

Use your Eating Profile to help you develop more effective eating patterns.

Learning how to "eat to live" sometimes requires new thinking:

Once there was an egg and it hatched.
Out popped a chick . . .
Along came a big bad wolf.
So . . . the chick *unhatched*!

Think before you eat . . .
Plan before you eat.

HUNGER NOT APPETITE

I "eat to live" . . . I eat because I'm hungry.

Sometimes I eat because I'm upset.
When I'm upset, I can substitute . . .

low calorie foods: carrot "chips" (or coins)
herbal teas
decaffeinated espresso
mineral water

physical activities: walk briskly out of the kitchen
walk briskly outside
walk briskly inside
climb the stairs
climb into bed

Add your own special ideas . . . use your wonderful imagination!

Think before you eat . . .
Plan before you eat.

Eating can be an emotional experience . . .

When I scraped my knee, I got a lollipop.

When I went to the doctor, I got a lollipop.

When I went to the dentist, I got a lollipop.

When I visited Grandma, I got a lollipop or a cookie.

This happened long ago . . . but I remember.
I remember . . . and now I understand.

Think before you eat . . .
Plan before you eat.

Some "food for thought" . . .

"Clean your plate."
"Clean your plate because of the starving people in Africa."
"Clean your plate because of the starving people in India."
"Clean your plate so you can have dessert!"

Now I'm learning to put less on my plate . . .

Think before you eat . . .
Plan before you eat.

Some more "food for thought" . . .

A calorie is a calorie . . . is a calorie.

It just takes many many more mouthfuls of salad to equal the calories in a brownie!

I can eat:

25 chocolate chip cookies and 2 cucumber slices, or
25 cucumber slices and 0 chocolate chip cookies, or
25 cucumber slices and 2 chocolate chip cookies!

I can eat:

25 potato chips and 3 celery sticks, or
25 celery sticks and 0 potato chips, or
25 celery sticks and 5 potato chips.

Yes, you can eat *just* five!

NOW WRITE YOUR OWN EQUATIONS!!

Think before you eat . . .
Plan before you eat.

"MAINTENANCE MATH"

Weight Management = Food Management — Prolonged Satisfaction
Weight Management = Food Management — Ongoing Satisfaction

Controlled Eating = Portion Control

Large portions of low calorie foods = Weight Loss Maintenance
Large portions of high calorie foods = Weight Gain
Small portions of high calorie foods = Weight Control

Portion Control ⟶ Weight Control
Weight Control ⟶ Prolonged Satisfaction
Weight Control ⟶ Ongoing Satisfaction

"TAKE A TASTE" ⟶ Weight Control
"TAKE A TASTE" ⟶ Prolonged Satisfaction
"TAKE A TASTE" ⟶ Ongoing Satisfaction

Think before you eat . . .
Plan before you eat.

DIRECTED EATING

Directed eating is controlled eating.
Directed eating is not deprived eating.
Directed eating can be ongoing.

Some foods are more desirable than other foods.
Some foods are more empowering . . .

There are no forbidden foods on a maintenance diet . . .

Controlled eating is not only part of weight loss
Controlled eating is part of maintenance . . .
Controlled eating is a part of life.

Controlled eating can be ongoing . . .
Controlled eating can produce prolonged satisfaction.

Directed eating is empowering . . .
Maintenance eating is empowering!
Controlled eating is empowering!

Think before you eat . . .
Plan before you eat.

"I WANT"

"I want to control my weight."
"I want to control my weight every day of my life."

"I want to maintain my weight."
"I want to maintain my weight every day of my life."

I think before I eat . . .
I plan before I eat . . .

This maintenance handbook is designed for the educated dieter!

The effective dieter discovers . . .

Eating habits
Eating preferences
Eating lifestyle

. . . and designs an Eating Profile.

The effective dieter keeps a daily record of what s/he eats.
The effective dieter takes control!

III

Weight Management Techniques

♦ · ♦ · ♦ · ♦ · ♦ · ♦ · ♦ · ♦ · ♦ · ♦ · ♦ · ♦ · ♦ · ♦ · ♦ · ♦ · ♦ · ♦ · ♦

Once there was an *effective eater.* S/he modified her/his everyday eating. And when s/he practiced a more flexible approach to dieting, s/he discovered JOY—the joy of eating, the joy of being in control, the joy of feeling and looking good!

♦ · ♦ · ♦ · ♦ · ♦ · ♦ · ♦ · ♦ · ♦ · ♦ · ♦ · ♦ · ♦ · ♦ · ♦ · ♦ · ♦ · ♦ · ♦

The ***effective eater*** plans . . .

REFOCUSING

Write down your *Daily Diet Plan:*

Choose your "weight mode" . . . "I want to lose weight today."
"I want to gain weight today."
"I want to maintain weight today."

Pre-plan your menu considering . . .

FOOD SELECTION

PORTION CONTROL

Remember to include your

ACTIVITY LEVEL

Refer to your Eating Profile.

Allow for the unexpected, especially if you're going out to eat.

Think positive!

WEIGHT MANAGEMENT

FOOD SELECTION	PORTION CONTROL	ACTIVITY LEVEL

determine

my daily weight mode:

WEIGHT LOSS?
WEIGHT GAIN?
WEIGHT MAINTENANCE?

PRE-PLANNING

Pre-plan your menu before going to . . . parties
restaurants
business luncheons
holiday feasts
birthday celebrations
anniversary celebrations
family reunions
vacations . . .

Write down the foods you plan to eat.
Write down the amounts.
Write down possible changes or substitutions.

At buffets "TAKE A TASTE" of most foods . . .
A "taste" = 2 tablespoons or less.

Be prepared . . . discover a new flexibility!

PRE-PLANNING FOR SPECIAL OCCASIONS

Choose your weight mode . . .
    I want to maintain my weight . . .

"Eat lean" during the week(s) preceding the event . . .
    (If weekends are special events "eat lean" during the week.)

Portion control = Directed eating
    Directed eating = Control

Portion control = The bridge between weight loss and maintenance . . .

Portion control = won't power
will power
self control
true *self* control

A sense of direction gives you control.

The *effective eater* asks,
"What is the *cost* of putting this in my mouth?"

SAMPLE MENUS*

Thanksgiving Dinner

Vegetable appetizers—all I want
1 cup consomme
2 slices turkey, white meat
½ cup stuffing
"taste" (1 tbsp.) mashed potatoes
"taste" (1 tbsp.) sweet potatoes
1 cup green beans (no butter)
½ cup brocolli
½ cup corn
cranberry sauce—not worth the calories
1 slice pumpkin pie with "taste" (2 tbsp.) whipped cream spread across top
1 glass wine
Coffee

Vacation: Day #1 (Restaurant)

1 Mai Tai (maybe two)
Grilled fish
1 cup steamed vegetables
Large salad
Dessert (split?)
2 glasses wine (*if* one Mai Tai)

*These pre-planned menus are maintenance menus.
Menus can likewise be planned for weight gain and weight loss.

PORTION CONTROL

"Sugar Control"

Split a dessert . . .
Share a banana split . . .
Nibble a petit-four
Order a one-scoop sundae
Special ice creams are worth the cost . . . unless you prefer "crunchies" . . .

"Count your Crunchies"

Count your corn chips
Count your potato chips
Count your peanuts
Count your pretzel sticks
Count your chocolate-covered macadamia nuts . . .

Order an appetizer instead of an entree . . .
Share an entree . . .

The *effective eater* asks,
"What is the *cost* of putting this in my mouth?"

"TAKE A TASTE"

. . . a portion of high calorie food during a weight-loss diet
. . . a portion of high calorie food during maintenance
. . . a portion at a buffet
. . . a portion at a wine tasting
. . . a portion at a wine and cheese party
. . . a portion at a dessert party

The first bite will make me happy.
The first taste is the best taste.
The second taste is delicious, too.

I don't have to eat the whole thing!
I don't have to eat the whole pizza!
I don't have to eat the whole cream puff!

Nothing tastes as good as being slim feels
. . . nothing!

CUT 'N SHOVE

How to Handle Oversize Restaurant Portions

One forkful into your mouth . . .
one forkful to the back of your plate.

Alternate these two steps when necessary.

Cha-Cha-Cha!!

Redesign Your Eating World

We learn new behavior in small steps . . .
Successful small steps give us a sense of encouragement.
Small achievements are the building blocks of success . . .

Ever learn to ice skate?
Ever build a bridge?

Ever learn to knit a sweater?
Ever learn to ski?

Ever climb a mountain?
Ever ride a train?

Ever climb a tree?
Ever climb aboard?

Ever paint a house?
Ever paint a picture of a house?

Ever plant a garden?
Ever build a sand castle?

The *effective eater* plans . . . his or her eating world!

Success *Can* Be Repeated . . .

If you lose only five pounds this year,
And keep it off . . .
consider it a success!

If you lose only ten pounds this year,
and keep it off . . .
consider it a success!

If you maintain any weight loss this year . . .
consider it a cause for celebration!

"Once upon a time there was a man who used portion control . . .
he considered his eating life a success!"

The *effective eater* plans consciously!

EATING ASSERTIVENESS

The right to say "No" . . . to food
The right to say "Yes" . . . to food

ANSWER: "NOT RIGHT NOW, MAYBE LATER."
QUESTION: WHAT DO YOU SAY TO AUNT MILLIE WHEN SHE OFFERS YOU HER SWEET POTATO PIE?

Affirm yourself!! Enjoy yourself!!

The *effective eater* plans . . . assertively!

THINK SLIM!

Replace eating as a pastime. . .

EXERCISE!

Go for a walk . . .
Go for a run . . .

Go to the movies . . .
Go to the beach . . .

Go to bed . . .
Go fly a kite . . .

GO FOR IT!

Nothing tastes as good as being slim feels
. . . nothing!

IMAGING

Picture yourself on a sunlit beach . . .

You're wearing your favorite swimsuit
(or nothing at all) . . .

Caress your sleek body with suntan lotion.

A crowd gathers.

Now . . . hear the applause!

The *effective eater* images . . .

IMAGING

See yourself on a sparkling ski slope . . .

You're wearing your designer outfit.

Breathe in the exhilarating air . . .

Take off . . . to the nearest chalet.

Enter the doorway . . .

Everyone turns.

See the admiring glances . . .

Hear the exclamations of approval!

MORE IMAGING

You can barely see your reflection in the steamy bathroom mirror.

Slowly the mist rises . . .

Eagerly you look at your taut, muscled body . . .

You chuckle with delight.

LOOK OUT WORLD!

CREATE YOUR OWN FANTASY . . .

Image yourself!
Image yourself every night before you go to sleep!

Picture yourself anywhere you want to be!
Picture yourself slim!

Write your own fantasies . . .
Isn't it fun? Aren't you pleased?

Fantasies have a way of coming true . . .

The *effective eater* images . . . every night!

Give yourself a present . . .
See a new you every day . . .
You feel wonderful!
You hear your own applause!

CONGRATULATIONS!

This maintenance manual is designed especially for the *effective eater*!

The *effective eater* discovers the joy of being slim . . . forever!

Give yourself a present . . .

A NEW YOU!